Coping with Asthma

A Practical Approach to Managing Symptoms and Triggers

Comprehensive Guide to Understanding Asthma Symptoms, Treatment Options, and Strategies for a Breath of Fresh Air and more

Graham Julian Oliver

Disclaimer

The information provided in **Coping with Asthma – A Practical Approach to Managing Symptoms and Triggers** is intended for general informational purposes only. While every effort has been made to ensure the accuracy of the content, the author and publisher make no guarantees regarding the completeness or reliability of the information contained within this book.

This book is not a substitute for professional medical advice, diagnosis, or treatment. Always seek the advice of your physician or other qualified health provider with any questions you may have regarding a medical condition, including asthma. Never disregard professional medical advice or delay in seeking it because of something you have read in this book.

The author does not endorse any specific individual, product, website, organization, or other names that may be referenced or mentioned in this book. All references are provided for informational purposes only, and the inclusion of any reference does not imply endorsement or recommendation.

The use of any information provided in this book is solely at your own risk. The author and publisher shall not be liable for any damages arising from the use or inability to use the information presented in this book.

By reading this book, you acknowledge that you have read, understood, and agreed to this disclaimer.

"Coping with Asthma – A Practical Approach to Managing Symptoms and Triggers" serves as an essential guide for individuals navigating the complexities of asthma management. Asthma is not just a chronic respiratory condition; it is a multifaceted challenge that affects millions worldwide. This comprehensive resource emphasizes the critical importance of understanding asthma—defining it clearly and elucidating its various types, including allergic and non-allergic forms. It highlights the vital role of effective management in enhancing the quality of life for those living with asthma.

Awareness of symptoms is crucial for timely intervention, and the book adeptly guides readers through recognizing these signs, emphasizing the need for a proactive approach. By embracing a holistic methodology that combines medication, lifestyle adjustments, and emotional support, readers are empowered to take control of their asthma. Understanding the symptoms, the triggers that can exacerbate them, and the role of inflammation are pivotal to this journey. The book discusses common misconceptions surrounding asthma, ensuring that readers are well-informed about when to seek emergency care and the significance of regular medical check-ups.

Identifying triggers is a critical aspect of managing asthma, and this guide provides an exhaustive overview of both environmental and emotional factors. From pollutants and allergens to weather-related challenges, the text equips readers with strategies to mitigate exposure to these triggers. The importance of maintaining a clean living environment and employing hypoallergenic products is underscored, alongside practical advice on recognizing personal triggers through journaling and monitoring air quality.

The treatment section of the book breaks down various medications, distinguishing between controllers and relievers, and explaining the proper use of inhalers. The role of corticosteroids and biologics is thoroughly explored, ensuring readers understand their treatment options. The emphasis on adherence to prescribed medications is particularly vital, as it can significantly influence overall asthma control. Moreover, the guide encourages readers to engage in regular medication reviews with healthcare providers to adapt their treatment plans effectively.

An asthma action plan is an indispensable tool, and this guide provides a detailed framework for creating one that is personalized to individual needs. By documenting symptoms and triggers and implementing peak flow monitoring, readers are encouraged to take an active role in their health management. The importance of sharing this plan with family, friends, and caregivers cannot be overstated, as a supportive network can significantly ease the burden of managing asthma, particularly for children who may need additional support in school settings.

Lifestyle modifications play a pivotal role in asthma management, and the book thoroughly explores the intersection of nutrition, exercise, and mental well-being. By advocating for a balanced diet rich in anti-inflammatory foods and omega-3 fatty acids, readers are guided toward dietary choices that can enhance respiratory health. The section on exercise promotes physical activity as beneficial, provided it is approached safely, with specific breathing techniques and suitable sports highlighted for individuals with asthma.

Additionally, the emotional aspect of living with asthma is addressed, offering strategies for coping with anxiety and stress, which can often accompany chronic health conditions.

In summary, "Coping with Asthma" is an invaluable resource that not only informs but also inspires. It invites readers to embrace their journey with asthma through effective management strategies, comprehensive education, and a proactive mindset. By providing a thorough exploration of symptoms, triggers, treatment options, and lifestyle modifications, this guide ultimately empowers individuals to lead fulfilling lives, breathing freely and confidently.

Table of Contents

Introduction

Definition of Asthma

Asthma is a chronic respiratory condition characterized by inflammation and narrowing of the airways, which can lead to difficulty breathing, coughing, wheezing, and shortness of breath. This condition can be triggered by various factors, including allergens, respiratory infections, exercise, and environmental pollutants. Understanding asthma is crucial for recognizing symptoms early and taking preventive measures.

When asthma symptoms occur, the airways become swollen and produce excess mucus, making it challenging to breathe. Asthma can affect individuals of all ages, but it often begins in childhood. Knowing how asthma manifests helps individuals and caregivers identify symptoms and seek appropriate treatment promptly.

Importance of Management

Effective management of asthma is essential for maintaining a good quality of life. By understanding triggers and symptoms, individuals can implement strategies to reduce asthma attacks and enhance daily functioning. Regular consultations with healthcare professionals can help patients develop personalized asthma action plans tailored to their specific needs.

Management may include using quick-relief medications for acute symptoms and long-term control medications to prevent attacks. Additionally, lifestyle changes, such as avoiding triggers and maintaining a healthy environment, play a crucial role in asthma management. By proactively addressing asthma, individuals can lead a more active and fulfilling life.

Getting Started with Your Journey

Recognizing Symptoms

Awareness of asthma symptoms is vital for effective management. Common signs include wheezing, shortness of breath, chest tightness, and persistent coughing, especially at night or early in the morning. Beginners should keep a symptom diary to track when symptoms occur, their severity, and any potential triggers. This information can be shared with healthcare providers to refine treatment strategies.

To recognize symptoms early, it's essential to understand individual variations. For example, some individuals may experience symptoms during physical activity or in response to allergens. Regular peak flow monitoring can also help detect changes in lung function, allowing for prompt action when asthma is worsening. When symptoms are recognized early, interventions can be more effective, reducing the risk of severe asthma attacks.

Embracing a Holistic Approach

Managing asthma effectively requires a holistic approach that combines medication, lifestyle changes, and support systems. Begin by following your healthcare provider's medication plan, which may include inhalers or other prescribed medications. It's crucial to use these as directed, ensuring that you have quick-relief medications on hand for emergencies and long-term control medications for daily management.

Lifestyle changes play a significant role in asthma management. This includes avoiding known triggers, such as tobacco smoke, strong odors, and allergens like pollen and dust. Regular exercise can improve lung function, but it should be approached cautiously—consider speaking with a doctor about an appropriate exercise regimen. Additionally, seeking support from asthma education programs or support groups can provide motivation and valuable tips for managing your condition more effectively.

CHAPTER 1:

Understanding Asthma

Overview of Asthma and Its Types

Asthma is a chronic respiratory condition characterized by inflammation and narrowing of the airways, leading to difficulty in breathing. There are two primary types: allergic and non-allergic asthma. Allergic asthma is triggered by allergens like pollen, dust mites, or pet dander, while non-allergic asthma can be triggered by factors such as stress, exercise, or changes in weather. Understanding these types helps in identifying effective management strategies.

Recognizing the type of asthma you or your loved one has can significantly influence treatment. For allergic asthma, avoiding known allergens is crucial, while for non-allergic asthma, managing environmental triggers and stress levels becomes essential. Knowing the type helps tailor a personal asthma management plan that addresses specific symptoms and triggers.

Common Symptoms: Wheezing, Coughing, Shortness of Breath

Common asthma symptoms include wheezing, coughing, and shortness of breath. Wheezing is a high-pitched whistling sound made when breathing, particularly during exhalation. Coughing, especially at night or early morning, is often a result of airway irritation. Shortness of breath can occur during physical activity or at rest, indicating that the airways are constricted.

To effectively manage these symptoms, individuals should keep track of their occurrences. Recognizing patterns in symptom flare-ups can help identify triggers and adjust daily routines accordingly. Utilizing rescue inhalers as prescribed can provide quick relief during an asthma attack, ensuring smoother breathing.

The Role of Inflammation in Asthma

Inflammation plays a central role in asthma, causing the airways to swell and produce excess mucus, which leads to restricted airflow. This inflammation can result from exposure to allergens, irritants, or respiratory infections, exacerbating asthma symptoms. Understanding this process is crucial for effective management and treatment.

To combat airway inflammation, corticosteroids are often prescribed as inhalers or oral medications. These medications help reduce swelling and prevent asthma attacks by controlling the underlying inflammation. Consistent use as directed can lead to improved airway function and fewer symptoms.

Factors Contributing to Asthma Attacks (Triggers)

Asthma attacks can be triggered by various environmental and lifestyle factors. Common triggers include allergens (like pollen and pet dander), irritants (such as smoke and strong odors), weather changes, respiratory infections, and physical activity. Identifying these triggers is essential for effective asthma management.

To minimize exposure to triggers, keep a diary of activities, environments, and symptoms. Implementing preventive measures, such as using air purifiers, avoiding smoking, and maintaining a clean living space, can significantly reduce the likelihood of an asthma attack. Discussing specific triggers with a healthcare provider can help develop a personalized avoidance strategy.

Genetic vs. Environmental Factors

Asthma can result from a combination of genetic predisposition and environmental influences. Genetic factors may include a family history of asthma or allergies, which increases the likelihood of developing the condition. Conversely, environmental factors, such as exposure to pollutants or allergens during childhood, can also play a critical role.

Understanding the interplay between genetics and environment is essential for prevention and management. Individuals with a family history of asthma should be proactive about minimizing exposure to potential triggers and may benefit from early intervention and education on asthma management.

How Asthma Is Diagnosed (Tests and Assessments)

Asthma diagnosis typically involves a combination of medical history, physical examination, and specific tests. Healthcare providers may conduct lung function tests, such as spirometry, to assess how well the lungs are working. Allergy tests may also be performed to identify potential triggers contributing to asthma symptoms.

When visiting a healthcare provider, be prepared to discuss symptoms, frequency of attacks, and any triggers you've identified. This information will assist in accurate diagnosis and the development of a tailored treatment plan. Follow-up visits may be necessary to monitor lung function and adjust treatment as needed.

Understanding Peak Flow Monitoring

Peak flow monitoring involves measuring how quickly air can be exhaled from the lungs, providing insight into asthma control. A peak flow meter is a portable device that can be used at home to assess lung function. Regular monitoring can help detect changes in airway responsiveness before symptoms worsen.

To use a peak flow meter, stand up straight, take a deep breath, and exhale forcefully into the device. Record the measurement and compare it to personal best values or asthma action plan guidelines. Tracking these numbers can help identify when to adjust medications or seek medical advice.

The Impact of Asthma on Daily Life

Asthma can significantly impact daily activities, including exercise, work, and social interactions. Individuals may find themselves avoiding certain activities or environments to prevent symptoms, leading to decreased quality of life. Understanding how asthma affects daily life is crucial for effective management.

To navigate these challenges, develop an individualized asthma management plan that incorporates medications, trigger avoidance strategies, and a clear understanding of when to seek help. Engaging in open conversations with family, friends, and coworkers about asthma can foster support and understanding in managing the condition.

The Importance of an Asthma Action Plan

An asthma action plan is a personalized, written document that outlines how to manage asthma symptoms, including daily management strategies and what to do during an asthma attack. It typically includes medication instructions, a list of triggers, and guidance on when to seek emergency care. Having a clear plan helps individuals respond effectively to their symptoms.

To create an asthma action plan, work with a healthcare provider to develop a comprehensive strategy tailored to individual needs. Regularly review and update the plan as symptoms or medications change. Keep copies accessible at home, school, or work, ensuring that caregivers and teachers understand the plan for prompt action.

Common Misconceptions about Asthma

There are many misconceptions surrounding asthma that can hinder effective management. For instance, some believe asthma is just a childhood condition, while others think it is merely a minor illness. These misconceptions can prevent individuals from seeking necessary treatment or adhering to prescribed management strategies.

Education is key to dispelling these myths. Sharing accurate information about asthma with patients and their families can empower them to take charge of their health. Encourage open discussions with healthcare providers to address any misconceptions and ensure proper understanding of the condition and its management.

When to Seek Emergency Care

Knowing when to seek emergency care is vital for individuals with asthma. Signs of a severe asthma attack include difficulty speaking, blue lips or face, and persistent wheezing or coughing despite using a rescue inhaler. If symptoms do not improve with medication, emergency medical help is required.

To ensure safety, communicate with family members or friends about these warning signs. Having a plan in place for emergencies, including knowing the nearest medical facilities and how to contact emergency services, can make a critical difference during a severe asthma episode.

Importance of Regular Medical Check-Ups

Regular medical check-ups are essential for effective asthma management. These visits allow healthcare providers to assess lung function, review medication efficacy, and update asthma action plans. Regular assessments help track progress and identify potential issues before they escalate.

To maximize the benefits of check-ups, prepare a list of questions or concerns to discuss with your healthcare provider. Keeping track of symptoms and medication use between appointments can provide valuable information to tailor treatment and ensure optimal asthma control.

Resources for Further Education

There are numerous resources available for individuals seeking to learn more about asthma management. Websites like the American Lung Association and the Asthma and Allergy Foundation of America offer educational materials, tips, and support for patients and their families. Local support groups and asthma clinics can also provide valuable community resources.

Taking advantage of these resources can empower individuals with asthma to take control of their condition.

CHAPTER 2:

Identifying Triggers

Common Environmental Triggers (Pollution, Dust, Pollen)

Asthma can be significantly triggered by common environmental factors such as pollution, dust, and pollen. To manage these triggers, it's important to monitor local air quality reports and limit outdoor activities when pollution levels are high or pollen counts are elevated. Using air purifiers and regularly changing air filters in your home can also reduce the presence of these irritants.

Additionally, implementing a cleaning routine that includes dusting and vacuuming with HEPA filters will help minimize dust accumulation. Wearing a mask during high pollen seasons or when cleaning can further protect your lungs from irritants, making it easier to breathe comfortably.

Weather-Related Triggers (Cold Air, Humidity)

Weather conditions like cold air and high humidity can exacerbate asthma symptoms. To cope with cold air, wearing a scarf or a mask over your mouth and nose can help warm the air before it enters your lungs. Staying indoors during extreme weather conditions is also advisable, as this can minimize exposure to harsh environmental changes.

In humid conditions, using dehumidifiers indoors can help maintain optimal humidity levels, which should ideally be between 30-50%. Keeping windows closed during high humidity days can prevent damp air from entering your home, providing a more comfortable living environment for individuals with asthma.

Indoor Allergens (Pet Dander, Mold)

Indoor allergens such as pet dander and mold can trigger asthma symptoms in sensitive individuals. To manage pet dander, regular grooming of pets and maintaining a pet-free zone in the bedroom can significantly reduce exposure. Consider using HEPA vacuum cleaners and washing pet bedding frequently to keep dander levels low.

Mold thrives in damp areas, so it's essential to address any water leaks or humidity issues in your home. Regularly check areas such as bathrooms, basements, and kitchens for signs of mold growth and use mold-killing solutions to clean affected surfaces. Maintaining proper ventilation can also help prevent mold development.

Occupational Hazards (Fumes, Dust)

Many people are exposed to occupational hazards that can trigger asthma, such as fumes and dust. To minimize exposure at work, it's crucial to wear appropriate protective gear like masks or respirators in environments where these irritants are present. Speak with your employer about implementing safety measures to reduce exposure, such as improving ventilation or using less harmful materials.

If you know you are sensitive to specific chemicals or dust, discuss alternative roles or tasks that may limit your exposure. Taking breaks in clean air environments and utilizing equipment that reduces dust creation can also help manage symptoms effectively.

Emotional Triggers (Stress and Anxiety)

Stress and anxiety can significantly impact asthma symptoms, often leading to exacerbations. To manage these emotional triggers, consider practicing relaxation techniques such as deep breathing, meditation, or yoga, which can help reduce stress levels and promote overall well-being. Creating a daily routine that includes time for self-care and relaxation can also be beneficial.

It's important to recognize your emotional triggers and how they relate to your asthma symptoms. Keeping a journal to document instances of stress and their correlation with your asthma can provide valuable insights, helping you develop strategies to cope with anxiety and minimize its impact on your breathing.

Food-Related Triggers (Allergies)

Food allergies can also provoke asthma symptoms in some individuals. It's crucial to identify any specific food triggers through an elimination diet or allergy testing, which should be done under the guidance of a healthcare professional. Keep a food diary to track what you eat and any corresponding asthma symptoms, helping you pinpoint problematic foods.

Once identified, avoid these trigger foods entirely and educate yourself on reading food labels to ensure safety while dining out or shopping. Communicating your allergies to friends, family, and restaurant staff is also essential for preventing accidental exposure and maintaining control over your asthma.

The Impact of Exercise on Asthma

Exercise can be beneficial for individuals with asthma but can also act as a trigger in some cases. To safely incorporate exercise, start with low-intensity activities such as walking or swimming, and gradually increase the intensity as your body adapts. Always warm up before exercising to help your lungs adjust to physical activity and consider exercising indoors on days when pollen counts are high.

It's essential to consult with a healthcare provider to develop an exercise plan tailored to your needs. They may also recommend using a bronchodilator before physical activity to help prevent exercise-induced asthma symptoms, ensuring you can enjoy the benefits of staying active without compromising your health.

Recognizing Personal Triggers through Journaling

Journaling is a powerful tool for identifying personal asthma triggers. Keep a daily log of your symptoms, activities, and environmental conditions, noting any potential triggers you encounter. Over time, this record will help you recognize patterns and identify specific circumstances that lead to asthma flare-ups.

By understanding your unique triggers, you can make informed choices to avoid them. This proactive approach empowers you to manage your condition better and communicate effectively with your healthcare provider, ensuring you receive the best possible care tailored to your needs.

Strategies for Avoiding Triggers at Home

Creating a home environment that minimizes asthma triggers is essential for effective management. Start by reducing clutter, which can collect dust and allergens, and maintain a clean space through regular vacuuming and dusting. Designate certain areas as no-smoking zones and limit the use of strong cleaning products or air fresheners that can irritate your lungs.

Utilizing air purifiers with HEPA filters can significantly improve indoor air quality by removing allergens and irritants. Establishing a no-shoes policy indoors can also prevent the transfer of outdoor allergens, ensuring a safer, cleaner space to breathe freely.

Role of Air Quality and Ventilation

Air quality plays a crucial role in managing asthma symptoms. To maintain good air quality indoors, use exhaust fans in bathrooms and kitchens to eliminate moisture and reduce mold growth. Open windows when weather permits to allow fresh air circulation, but be mindful of outdoor pollen counts and air pollution levels.

Investing in an air quality monitor can help you stay informed about the indoor environment. When pollution levels are high, using an air purifier can help filter out harmful particles, providing cleaner air and reducing the likelihood of asthma attacks.

Importance of Regular Cleaning and Maintenance

Regular cleaning and maintenance of your home are vital in controlling asthma triggers. Establish a cleaning schedule that includes vacuuming, dusting, and washing bedding weekly to minimize allergens. Focus on high-risk areas such as carpets, upholstery, and curtains, as these can harbor dust mites and other irritants.

In addition to routine cleaning, regular maintenance of heating and cooling systems is crucial. Change filters according to the manufacturer's recommendations and have systems inspected annually to ensure optimal performance, helping to maintain a healthier indoor environment.

Use of Hypoallergenic Products

Using hypoallergenic products can significantly reduce exposure to allergens in your home. Look for cleaning supplies, laundry detergents, and personal care items labeled as hypoallergenic, as these are formulated to minimize irritants. It's also beneficial to choose furniture and bedding made from materials that are less likely to harbor allergens.

When shopping for hypoallergenic products, reading labels and reviews can help you make informed choices. Transitioning to these products can create a more asthma-friendly living space and contribute to overall respiratory health.

Testing for Specific Allergies

Testing for specific allergies is a crucial step in managing asthma effectively. Consult with an allergist to discuss your symptoms and undergo tests such as skin prick tests or blood tests to identify allergies. Understanding your specific triggers allows you to avoid them, reducing the risk of asthma exacerbations.

Once identified, it's essential to create a comprehensive plan that includes strategies to avoid allergens in your environment. Work closely with your healthcare provider to develop this plan, ensuring you have the resources and knowledge to manage your asthma effectively.

CHAPTER 3:

Medications and Treatment Options

Overview of Asthma Medications (Controllers vs. Relievers)

Asthma medications fall into two primary categories: controllers and relievers. Controllers, often taken daily, help prevent asthma symptoms by reducing inflammation in the airways and providing long-term control. These typically include inhaled corticosteroids, long-acting beta-agonists, and leukotriene modifiers. Relievers, on the other hand, are used for quick relief during an asthma attack or when symptoms flare up. They work by relaxing the muscles around the airways, allowing for easier breathing.

For effective asthma management, it's essential to understand the differences between these medications. Controllers should be taken consistently as prescribed to maintain lung health, while relievers should be on hand for unexpected symptoms. A balanced approach involving both types of medications can significantly improve overall asthma control and quality of life.

How Inhalers Work (MDI vs. Nebulizers)

Inhalers are devices that deliver medication directly to the lungs, and there are two main types: metered-dose inhalers (MDIs) and nebulizers. MDIs release a specific dose of medication as a mist, which you inhale. They are portable, easy to use, and ideal for quick relief. To maximize their effectiveness, it's crucial to use a spacer, which helps ensure that more medication reaches the lungs instead of being deposited in the mouth or throat.

Nebulizers, on the other hand, convert liquid medication into a fine mist that can be inhaled over a longer period. They are especially useful for individuals who struggle with using inhalers correctly or for young children. When using a nebulizer, make sure to follow the manufacturer's instructions on how to set it up and clean it properly to prevent infections.

Role of Corticosteroids in Asthma Management

Corticosteroids are a cornerstone of asthma management, particularly for controlling inflammation. These medications work by reducing swelling and mucus production in the airways, leading to improved breathing. They can be taken orally or through inhalation, with inhaled corticosteroids being preferred for long-term management due to fewer systemic side effects.

To effectively incorporate corticosteroids into your asthma plan, it's important to use them as prescribed and understand that they may take time to show benefits. Regular communication with your healthcare provider can help determine the right dosage and monitor any potential side effects.

Importance of Adherence to Prescribed Medications

Adherence to prescribed asthma medications is critical for effective management. Missing doses or discontinuing medication can lead to worsened symptoms and increased risk of asthma attacks. Establishing a routine, such as taking medications at the same time each day, can help ensure consistent use

To support adherence, consider using reminders through apps, alarms, or pill organizers. Engaging with your healthcare provider to discuss any concerns about medications can also help reinforce the importance of sticking to your treatment plan, making adjustments if necessary.

Understanding Long-Term vs. Short-Term Medications

Asthma management often involves both long-term and short-term medications. Long-term medications, like inhaled corticosteroids, are taken daily to maintain control over asthma symptoms. They reduce inflammation and prevent the occurrence of asthma attacks. Short-term medications, or rescue inhalers, provide immediate relief during sudden symptoms or attacks.

Recognizing when to use each type of medication is key. Ensure you have a long-term plan in place and use your rescue inhaler only when necessary. Discuss your medication regimen with your healthcare provider to ensure it aligns with your specific asthma management needs.

How to Use Inhalers Correctly (Technique)

Proper inhaler technique is vital for maximizing medication delivery to the lungs. Start by shaking the inhaler, then attach a spacer if you have one. Take a deep breath and exhale fully before placing the inhaler in your mouth. Press down on the inhaler while inhaling slowly and deeply, holding your breath for about 10 seconds afterward to allow the medication to settle.

Practicing this technique regularly can enhance its effectiveness. If using a nebulizer, ensure the machine is set up correctly and breathe normally until all the medication is used. Regular practice and checking your technique with your healthcare provider can help ensure you're using your inhaler effectively.

Side Effects of Common Asthma Medications

Like all medications, asthma treatments can have side effects. Common side effects of inhaled corticosteroids include a sore throat, oral thrush, and hoarseness. Short-acting bronchodilators may cause jitteriness or a rapid heartbeat. Understanding these potential side effects is essential for managing your treatment effectively.

To mitigate side effects, practice good inhaler hygiene, such as rinsing your mouth after using inhaled corticosteroids. If you experience persistent or severe side effects, consult your healthcare provider for potential alternatives or adjustments to your treatment plan.

The Role of Biologics in Severe Asthma Cases

Biologics are advanced treatments designed for individuals with severe asthma that does not respond well to standard therapies. These medications target specific pathways involved in the inflammatory response, offering a more tailored approach to treatment. Biologics can significantly reduce the frequency of asthma exacerbations and the need for oral corticosteroids.

For those considering biologics, a discussion with a healthcare provider is crucial to evaluate eligibility and understand the potential benefits and risks. Regular follow-ups are also important to monitor effectiveness and adjust treatment as necessary.

Understanding the Importance of Rescue Inhalers

Rescue inhalers are essential for managing acute asthma symptoms and attacks. These short-acting bronchodilators provide immediate relief by relaxing the airway muscles, allowing for easier breathing. It's crucial to always carry a rescue inhaler and know how to use it properly, as this can be life-saving in emergencies.

To ensure its effectiveness, check the expiration date regularly and replace it as needed. Familiarize yourself with your asthma action plan, which outlines when to use your rescue inhaler and when to seek emergency help.

Dosage and Timing for Optimal Effectiveness

Correct dosage and timing of asthma medications are essential for effective management. Long-term medications should be taken consistently as prescribed, while rescue inhalers should be used at the onset of symptoms. Understanding the specific timing for each medication can enhance their effectiveness.

Keep a medication log to track dosages and timing, which can also help identify patterns in symptom management. Discuss any adjustments with your healthcare provider to find the best regimen for your needs.

The Need for Regular Medication Reviews with Healthcare Providers

Regular medication reviews with healthcare providers are vital for optimizing asthma management. These reviews allow for adjustments based on the effectiveness of current treatments and any changes in symptoms. Engaging in these discussions can help ensure that you are using the most appropriate medications for your asthma type and severity.

During your review, be prepared to discuss your medication adherence, any side effects experienced, and any recent changes in your symptoms or triggers. This open communication can lead to better asthma control and an overall improved quality of life.

Exploring Alternative Treatments and Therapies

While conventional asthma medications are effective, some individuals seek alternative treatments and therapies. These may include herbal remedies, acupuncture, or breathing exercises. It's essential to approach these alternatives with caution and consult your healthcare provider before incorporating them into your asthma management plan.

Understanding that alternative treatments should complement, not replace, prescribed medications is crucial. Always prioritize evidence-based treatments and ensure that any new therapies align with your overall asthma strategy.

Importance of Emergency Medication Accessibility

Ensuring that emergency medication, such as rescue inhalers, is easily accessible is critical for managing asthma effectively. Keep a rescue inhaler in places you frequent, such as your home, car, and workplace. Inform those around you about your asthma and how they can assist in case of an emergency.

Regularly check the expiration dates of your rescue inhalers and ensure they are in working condition. Developing an asthma action plan with your healthcare provider can help clarify steps to take in an emergency, ensuring you are prepared for any situation.

CHAPTER 4:

Creating an Asthma Action Plan

Components of an Asthma Action Plan (Personalized Approach)

An asthma action plan is a personalized document that outlines your asthma management strategies, including medication dosages, triggers, and how to handle symptoms. Start by consulting your healthcare provider to include information such as the names of medications, when to take them, and how to recognize worsening symptoms. Make sure the plan is clear and easy to follow, incorporating visual aids if necessary to simplify the information.

Your action plan should be divided into three main sections: daily management, recognizing worsening symptoms, and emergency responses. Ensure it includes personalized peak flow meter readings, allowing you to monitor your lung function. Share your plan with family, friends, and caregivers to ensure everyone is aware of your specific needs and how to help during an asthma episode.

Importance of Documenting Symptoms and Triggers

Keeping a record of your asthma symptoms and potential triggers is essential for effective management. Maintain a daily journal where you note the frequency and severity of your symptoms, along with possible environmental or emotional triggers, such as pollen, smoke, or stress. This documentation helps you and your healthcare provider identify patterns and adjust treatment plans accordingly.

Utilize this information to discuss your experiences during medical appointments. By presenting detailed records, you can help your provider tailor your medication and management strategies more effectively. A symptom diary also empowers you to take proactive steps in avoiding known triggers, ultimately reducing the risk of asthma flare-ups.

Setting Up Peak Flow Monitoring

Peak flow monitoring is a valuable tool for tracking your asthma control. To set it up, obtain a peak flow meter, a handheld device that measures how well air moves out of your lungs. Begin by establishing your personal best peak flow reading when your asthma is well-controlled, ideally in the morning before taking medication.

Once you have your baseline, use the meter regularly (at least once daily) and note the readings. Record the results in a chart, noting any factors that may influence the readings, such as weather or activities. This monitoring enables you to identify early warning signs of worsening asthma and take appropriate action according to your asthma action plan.

Identifying Zones (Green, Yellow, Red)

Identifying zones in your asthma action plan helps categorize your symptoms and peak flow readings into three distinct levels: green, yellow, and red. The green zone indicates good control, where symptoms are minimal, and peak flow readings are at or above 80% of your personal best. In this zone, continue your usual management routine.

The yellow zone signals caution, indicating that your asthma may be worsening. Here, symptoms may increase, and peak flow readings drop to 50-79% of your personal best. In this case, follow the instructions in your action plan, which may include using a quick-relief inhaler or adjusting medications. The red zone represents a medical emergency, where peak flow readings are below 50% of your personal best, requiring immediate action and possibly emergency medical assistance.

Steps to Take During an Asthma Attack

During an asthma attack, stay calm and follow your asthma action plan. Immediately use your quick-relief inhaler as prescribed. If you experience severe symptoms—such as difficulty speaking, wheezing, or chest tightness—seek help from someone nearby. Sit up straight to facilitate easier breathing and try to relax as much as possible.

If symptoms do not improve within a few minutes after using your inhaler, take your rescue medication again as directed. If you are still struggling to breathe, contact emergency services or go to the nearest hospital. Remember to keep your action plan accessible and communicate your situation clearly to others who may assist you during the attack.

How to Communicate Your Action Plan with Others

Effectively communicating your asthma action plan with family, friends, and caregivers is vital for ensuring support during an emergency. Schedule a time to share the plan, making sure to explain the various components, including how to recognize symptoms and the appropriate actions to take in each zone. Use simple language and encourage questions to clarify any uncertainties.

In addition to verbal communication, consider sharing a copy of your action plan with those who may be involved in your care, such as school staff or coworkers. This ensures everyone is on the same page and can act quickly if needed. Regularly remind them about the importance of being prepared and how they can assist in case of an asthma attack.

Regularly Reviewing and Updating Your Action Plan

Your asthma action plan should not be static; it requires regular reviews and updates. Schedule periodic check-ins with your healthcare provider, especially after experiencing changes in symptoms or medication adjustments. Use these meetings to evaluate the effectiveness of your current management strategies and make necessary adjustments based on your experiences and peak flow readings.

Updating your action plan ensures it remains relevant and effective. Keep a copy handy and revisit it frequently, especially during seasonal changes or after significant life events that may affect your asthma, such as moving to a new area or starting a new job.

The Role of Healthcare Providers in Your Plan

Healthcare providers play a crucial role in developing and maintaining your asthma action plan. They offer expert guidance on medication management, inhaler techniques, and recognizing symptoms. During your appointments, be open about your experiences, challenges, and any concerns you have regarding your asthma. This information allows your provider to tailor your plan effectively.

Regular communication with your healthcare provider ensures you receive timely updates on new treatments or strategies. They can also assist you in identifying additional resources, such as support groups or educational materials, to further enhance your understanding and management of asthma.

Involving Family and Friends in Your Management

Involving family and friends in your asthma management fosters a supportive environment. Start by educating them about your condition, explaining how asthma affects you, and what triggers your symptoms. Encourage open dialogue about your experiences, so they can better understand your needs and respond appropriately during an asthma attack.

In addition to education, involve them in your daily asthma management routine. Encourage family members to help you keep track of your medications and symptoms, and practice inhaler techniques together. This collaboration not only enhances your support system but also helps reduce feelings of isolation associated with managing a chronic condition.

Strategies for Children and School Environments

Managing asthma in children requires a tailored approach, especially in school settings. Start by communicating with school staff about your child's condition and ensure they have access to their medication. Provide teachers and school nurses with a copy of your child's asthma action plan and educate them on recognizing symptoms and appropriate responses.

Implement strategies to help your child identify and avoid triggers at school, such as keeping their environment free from allergens and ensuring a smoke-free space. Encourage open discussions with your child about their asthma, empowering them to advocate for themselves and communicate their needs effectively with peers and adults.

Emergency Contacts and Procedures

Establishing a list of emergency contacts and procedures is critical for effective asthma management. Include family members, friends, and healthcare providers who can assist in a crisis. Ensure that this list is easily accessible, perhaps posted in a common area at home or saved in your phone for quick reference.

In addition to contacts, outline clear emergency procedures. This includes what to do in case of an asthma attack, when to call for help, and what information to provide to emergency responders. Regularly review and practice these procedures with family and friends to ensure everyone knows their role during an asthma crisis.

Importance of Carrying a Written Plan

Carrying a written asthma action plan is vital for quick reference during emergencies. Always keep a copy in your bag, car, or other easily accessible locations. A written plan can guide you through various situations, particularly if you are in an unfamiliar environment or when someone unfamiliar with your condition is assisting you.

In addition to your written plan, consider carrying an emergency card that summarizes your critical information, such as medications, dosages, and emergency contacts. This card can be especially helpful during travel or outings, ensuring that you have vital information at hand when needed.

Utilizing Mobile Apps for Tracking

Mobile apps can significantly enhance your asthma management by providing tools for tracking symptoms, medications, and peak flow readings. Start by selecting an app that suits your needs, ensuring it allows for easy input of data and offers reminders for medication and peak flow monitoring. Many apps also provide educational resources and tips for managing asthma effectively.

Regularly input your symptoms and peak flow data into the app to identify patterns over time. Use the insights gained from this tracking to discuss with your healthcare provider during appointments, allowing for more informed decisions about your asthma management strategies. Mobile apps can empower you to take a proactive approach to your asthma care.

CHAPTER 5:

Lifestyle Modifications

The Role of Nutrition in Asthma Management

Nutrition plays a critical role in managing asthma symptoms and overall lung health. A balanced diet rich in fruits, vegetables, whole grains, and lean proteins provides essential nutrients that support the immune system and reduce inflammation. Incorporating foods high in antioxidants, such as berries, leafy greens, and nuts, can help combat oxidative stress, which may trigger asthma attacks.

Additionally, certain nutrients like omega-3 fatty acids found in fish and flaxseed have anti-inflammatory properties that can benefit asthma sufferers. It is essential to identify and avoid food allergens that may exacerbate symptoms, such as dairy or sulfites. Keeping a food diary can help track what you eat and its impact on your asthma, allowing for better dietary choices.

Benefits of Regular Exercise (Breathing Techniques)

Regular exercise is beneficial for individuals with asthma as it can enhance lung function and reduce the frequency of asthma attacks. Activities like walking, swimming, or cycling help improve cardiovascular fitness and strengthen respiratory muscles. Incorporating breathing techniques, such as diaphragmatic breathing and pursed-lip breathing, during exercise can further promote better oxygen flow and help manage shortness of breath.

To start, engage in moderate activities for 20-30 minutes, several times a week, and gradually increase intensity as tolerated. It's crucial to warm up before exercising and cool down afterward, allowing your body to adjust and prevent asthma symptoms. Always consult a healthcare provider before starting any new exercise program, especially if your asthma is not well controlled.

Maintaining a Healthy Weight for Asthma Control

Maintaining a healthy weight is essential for effective asthma management, as obesity can worsen symptoms and increase the risk of complications. Excess weight places additional strain on the lungs, making it harder to breathe. A balanced diet combined with regular physical activity is the best approach to achieving and sustaining a healthy weight.

To manage your weight, focus on portion control, eating nutrient-dense foods, and incorporating physical activities you enjoy into your daily routine. Consulting a nutritionist can provide personalized meal plans and tips tailored to your needs, ensuring you lose weight healthily without triggering asthma symptoms.

Importance of Hydration

Staying well-hydrated is vital for individuals with asthma, as dehydration can lead to increased mucus production, making it more challenging to breathe. Drinking enough water helps maintain proper lung function and supports overall health. Aim to consume at least eight 8-ounce glasses of water daily, adjusting for factors such as exercise, climate, and personal needs.

In addition to plain water, consider incorporating herbal teas or broths to enhance hydration. Avoid excessive caffeine and alcohol, as they can lead to dehydration. Keeping a water bottle handy throughout the day can serve as a reminder to drink more fluids and stay hydrated.

Strategies for Stress Management (Mindfulness, Relaxation)

Managing stress is crucial for asthma control, as stress can trigger symptoms or exacerbate existing conditions. Practicing mindfulness techniques, such as meditation, yoga, or deep breathing exercises, can help reduce anxiety and improve your ability to cope with stressors. Regularly setting aside time for these practices can promote relaxation and enhance overall well-being.

To incorporate mindfulness into your daily routine, start with just a few minutes each day and gradually increase the duration. You can also join local classes or use smart phone apps that provide guided sessions to help you stay on track. Establishing a consistent practice will not only benefit your mental health but may also lead to fewer asthma-related issues.

Importance of Sleep and Its Impact on Asthma

Quality sleep is essential for everyone, but particularly for individuals with asthma, as sleep deprivation can worsen symptoms and decrease overall health. Poor sleep can lead to increased inflammation and weakened immune response, making asthma attacks more likely. Aim for 7-9 hours of uninterrupted sleep each night to promote better respiratory health.

To improve sleep quality, create a relaxing bedtime routine and maintain a consistent sleep schedule. Ensure your sleeping environment is comfortable, cool, and free from allergens, such as dust mites or pet dander. If sleep apnea or other sleep disorders are suspected, consult a healthcare professional for proper evaluation and management.

Quitting Smoking and Avoiding Secondhand Smoke

Quitting smoking is one of the most effective steps individuals can take to improve asthma management. Smoking irritates the airways, increases inflammation, and heightens the risk of severe asthma attacks. If you smoke, seek help from healthcare providers, support groups, or cessation programs to create a tailored quitting plan that suits your needs.

Avoiding secondhand smoke is equally important, as it can exacerbate asthma symptoms in sensitive individuals. Advocate for smoke-free environments at home, work, and public places. Encourage friends and family to respect your asthma by refraining from smoking around you, ensuring you can breathe easier.

How to Prepare for Seasonal Changes

Seasonal changes can impact asthma symptoms, making it essential to prepare in advance. Keep track of pollen counts, weather changes, and temperature fluctuations to anticipate potential triggers. During high pollen seasons, stay indoors when possible, keep windows closed, and use air conditioning to filter outdoor air.

Additionally, consider adjusting your medication regimen as the seasons change. Consult with your healthcare provider to create an action plan for managing asthma during seasonal transitions. Keeping your home environment clean, using air purifiers, and regularly changing HVAC filters can also help mitigate triggers related to seasonal changes.

Tips for Traveling with Asthma (Medication Storage)

Traveling with asthma requires careful planning to ensure you have access to your medications and avoid potential triggers. Always carry a sufficient supply of your inhalers and medications, ideally in their original packaging, along with a copy of your prescriptions. It's advisable to keep these in your carry-on bag to prevent loss or damage during transit.

When traveling, familiarize yourself with the locations of hospitals or clinics in your destination area in case of an emergency. Pack a small travel kit with your inhaler, spacer, and any necessary medications. If traveling by air, check airline regulations for carrying medications and inquire about in-flight accommodations for asthma.

Adapting Hobbies and Activities to Fit Your Condition

Adapting hobbies and activities to suit your asthma condition can ensure you stay active without triggering symptoms. For instance, consider low-impact activities such as walking, swimming, or yoga, which are generally easier on the lungs. If you enjoy outdoor activities, choose times when pollen counts are lower or opt for indoor alternatives when necessary.

Always listen to your body and adjust your activities based on how you feel. For instance, if you notice certain hobbies trigger your asthma, find modifications or alternatives that allow you to enjoy those activities safely. Keeping an open dialogue with family and friends can also help them understand your needs and support you in your hobbies.

Seeking Support Groups or Community Resources

Joining support groups or utilizing community resources can significantly aid in managing asthma. Connecting with others who share similar experiences can provide emotional support, practical advice, and valuable coping strategies. Many organizations offer local or online support groups, allowing you to share your journey and learn from others.

Additionally, community resources like asthma education programs, workshops, and health fairs can provide essential information on managing asthma. Participating in these activities can enhance your understanding of asthma and empower you to take control of your health effectively.

The Importance of Education for Family Members

Educating family members about asthma is crucial for creating a supportive environment. Ensure they understand the condition, triggers, and emergency procedures, enabling them to assist you during asthma attacks or manage your condition effectively. Providing resources, such as pamphlets or websites, can help them grasp the seriousness of asthma and how to offer support.

Regular family discussions about asthma management can foster a collaborative approach to coping strategies and daily routines. Encouraging family members to participate in your asthma care can enhance their awareness and commitment to maintaining a safe environment, ultimately leading to better asthma control.

Utilizing Technology for Monitoring and Support

Technology can play a significant role in managing asthma, offering tools for monitoring symptoms and accessing support. Smartphone apps can help track medication usage, peak flow readings, and environmental triggers, providing valuable insights into your condition. Regularly reviewing this data can help you and your healthcare provider make informed decisions about your asthma management plan.

Additionally, online platforms and forums offer opportunities to connect with others living with asthma, sharing experiences and advice. Telehealth services can also facilitate remote consultations with healthcare providers, making it easier to manage your asthma and stay on top of your treatment plan.

CHAPTER 6:

Nutrition and Asthma

The Link between Diet and Asthma Symptoms

Diet plays a crucial role in managing asthma symptoms, as certain foods can exacerbate or alleviate respiratory issues. For instance, processed foods high in sugar and unhealthy fats may trigger inflammation, while a diet rich in whole foods can help support lung function. To manage asthma effectively, it is essential to be aware of how different foods affect your body and symptoms.

By focusing on a balanced diet that includes fruits, vegetables, whole grains, and lean proteins, individuals can create a nutritional foundation that may help minimize asthma symptoms. Keeping track of any changes in symptoms related to dietary changes is also vital to identifying personal triggers and making necessary adjustments.

Foods That May Help Reduce Inflammation

Incorporating anti-inflammatory foods into your diet can be a practical way to reduce asthma symptoms. Foods such as berries, leafy greens, and fatty fish are known for their anti-inflammatory properties. These foods can help lower the body's inflammatory response, potentially leading to improved lung function and reduced asthma attacks.

To maximize the benefits, aim to include a variety of these foods in your daily meals. For example, try a breakfast smoothie with spinach and blueberries or a lunch featuring grilled salmon with a side of kale salad. This approach can help ensure that you receive a range of nutrients essential for respiratory health.

Importance of Omega-3 Fatty Acids

Omega-3 fatty acids, found in fatty fish, flaxseeds, and walnuts, are essential for reducing inflammation and improving lung health. These healthy fats can help decrease the severity of asthma symptoms by modulating inflammatory processes in the body. Incorporating omega-3-rich foods into your diet can be a simple yet effective strategy for asthma management.

To add more omega-3s to your meals, consider swapping out traditional cooking oils for flaxseed oil or adding a serving of walnuts to your salad. Consuming fatty fish, like salmon or mackerel, at least twice a week can also significantly boost your omega-3 intake.

Identifying Food Allergens and Sensitivities

Understanding food allergens and sensitivities is crucial for managing asthma symptoms effectively. Common allergens like dairy, nuts, and gluten can trigger asthma attacks in sensitive individuals. The first step is to identify which foods may be causing adverse reactions by observing symptoms after consumption.

To pinpoint specific allergens, consider eliminating suspected foods from your diet for a few weeks and then reintroducing them one at a time. This process, known as an elimination diet, can help you determine which foods to avoid, allowing you to tailor your diet for better asthma control.

The Role of Antioxidants in Respiratory Health

Antioxidants play a significant role in protecting lung cells from oxidative stress, which can worsen asthma symptoms. Foods high in antioxidants, such as fruits, vegetables, nuts, and whole grains, help combat inflammation and support overall respiratory health. Incorporating a variety of colorful fruits and vegetables into your meals can maximize your antioxidant intake.

To boost your antioxidant consumption, aim to fill half your plate with fruits and vegetables at every meal. For example, snack on berries or carrot sticks, and enjoy salads made with a variety of colorful produce to enhance your lung health while adding flavor and nutrients to your diet.

Importance of Maintaining a Balanced Diet

Maintaining a balanced diet is vital for managing asthma symptoms effectively. A well-rounded diet provides essential nutrients that support lung function and overall health. Prioritizing a mix of carbohydrates, proteins, and healthy fats can help ensure your body has the resources it needs to function optimally.

To achieve a balanced diet, aim to include a variety of food groups in each meal. For instance, combine whole grains with lean protein and plenty of vegetables to create a nutritious dish. Planning meals ahead of time can help ensure that you are meeting your dietary needs consistently.

Hydration Tips for Optimal Lung Function

Staying properly hydrated is essential for optimal lung function, as it helps maintain the moisture in airways and supports overall respiratory health. Dehydration can lead to thicker mucus production, making it harder to breathe. Aim to drink plenty of water throughout the day to keep your body well-hydrated.

A practical tip for ensuring adequate hydration is to carry a water bottle with you at all times. Set reminders to drink water regularly, especially if you tend to forget. Additionally, consuming hydrating foods like cucumbers and watermelon can contribute to your overall fluid intake.

Exploring Anti-Inflammatory Diets

An anti-inflammatory diet focuses on reducing inflammation in the body, which can be particularly beneficial for asthma management. This type of diet emphasizes whole foods like fruits, vegetables, nuts, seeds, and lean proteins while minimizing processed foods and refined sugars. By prioritizing these foods, you can support your respiratory health.

To adopt an anti-inflammatory diet, begin by gradually replacing processed snacks with whole-food alternatives. For example, swap chips for a handful of nuts or replace sugary desserts with fresh fruit. Experimenting with different recipes and meal ideas can help you discover enjoyable ways to maintain this diet long-term.

The Impact of Obesity on Asthma Control

Obesity can significantly impact asthma control, as excess weight places additional strain on the respiratory system. It can lead to increased inflammation and reduce lung function, making it essential to manage body weight for optimal asthma management. A focus on healthy eating and regular physical activity can help in achieving and maintaining a healthy weight.

Start by setting realistic goals for weight management through small, sustainable changes in your diet and activity level. Consider incorporating more physical activity into your daily routine, such as walking or biking, while also making healthier food choices to support your weight loss efforts.

Strategies for Meal Planning and Preparation

Meal planning and preparation can help individuals manage their asthma symptoms by ensuring they have access to healthy, nourishing foods. Planning meals in advance allows you to make intentional food choices that align with your dietary needs. Start by dedicating time each week to outline meals and create a shopping list.

When preparing meals, focus on batch cooking and using fresh ingredients to minimize reliance on processed foods. Cooking larger portions can save time throughout the week and provide convenient options when you need them, helping you maintain a healthy diet without added stress.

Consulting with a Dietitian for Personalized Plans

Working with a registered dietitian can provide valuable insights into managing asthma through diet. A dietitian can help create a personalized meal plan based on your specific health needs, preferences, and any identified food sensitivities. This tailored approach can significantly improve your asthma management strategy.

During your consultation, be open about your symptoms and dietary habits to allow the dietitian to make informed recommendations. They can provide practical tips and resources to help you implement dietary changes effectively, empowering you to take charge of your asthma management.

Importance of Regular Meal Times and Balanced Nutrition

Establishing regular meal times can help regulate blood sugar levels and support overall health, which is particularly important for individuals managing asthma. Eating at consistent times throughout the day can also help prevent overeating and promote better food choices. Aim for three balanced meals and healthy snacks at regular intervals.

To maintain balanced nutrition, focus on including a variety of food groups in each meal. By ensuring that you have a good mix of proteins, healthy fats, and complex carbohydrates, you can support your body's needs while managing asthma symptoms more effectively.

Keeping a Food Diary for Tracking Reactions

Keeping a food diary is a practical tool for identifying food triggers and monitoring how your diet affects your asthma symptoms. By recording what you eat and any subsequent symptoms, you can identify patterns that may indicate food sensitivities or allergies. This process can be incredibly helpful for making informed dietary adjustments.

To start a food diary, keep it simple by noting the foods you consume and any symptoms experienced, including their timing and severity.

CHAPTER 7:

Exercise and Breathing Techniques

The Benefits of Exercise for Asthma Management

Exercise is essential for managing asthma as it strengthens the respiratory system and improves lung function. Regular physical activity helps reduce inflammation in the airways and enhances overall cardiovascular health, which can decrease asthma symptoms and frequency of attacks. Furthermore, exercise promotes the release of endorphins, which can improve mood and reduce stress, two common asthma triggers.

To maximize the benefits, aim for at least 150 minutes of moderate aerobic activity each week, such as walking, swimming, or cycling. Engaging in exercise not only builds endurance but also encourages better breathing patterns and helps individuals feel more in control of their asthma.

Safe Exercise Options for Asthma Patients

Asthma patients can safely engage in low to moderate-intensity exercises that minimize the risk of triggering symptoms. Activities like walking, cycling, and swimming are often recommended because they provide consistent airflow and are less likely to induce breathlessness. It is crucial to start gradually, allowing the body to adapt and monitoring how it reacts to different forms of exercise.

Before beginning a new exercise program, consult a healthcare provider for personalized recommendations and to ensure the chosen activities align with your specific asthma management plan. Always keep a rescue inhaler on hand in case of sudden symptoms while exercising.

Importance of Warm-Up and Cool-Down Routines

Incorporating warm-up and cool-down routines is vital for asthma patients, as these practices help prepare the body for exercise and promote recovery afterward. A proper warm-up gradually increases the heart rate and loosens the muscles, which can help minimize the risk of exercise-induced bronchoconstriction. This may include light stretching and low-intensity movements to ease into the workout.

After exercising, a cool-down period helps bring the heart rate back to normal and allows for controlled breathing. This period can involve gentle stretching and deep breathing exercises, helping to prevent post-exercise asthma symptoms and ensuring a smooth transition back to rest.

Breathing Techniques (Diaphragmatic Breathing)

Diaphragmatic breathing is a useful technique for asthma patients, allowing for more efficient lung use. This method involves breathing deeply through the nose, allowing the diaphragm to expand rather than just the chest, which can help improve oxygen intake and promote relaxation. To practice, find a comfortable position, place one hand on your chest and the other on your abdomen, and focus on moving your diaphragm while keeping your chest still.

Incorporate this technique into your daily routine, especially during times of increased stress or before exercising. Practicing diaphragmatic breathing regularly can enhance lung function, reduce anxiety, and lead to better overall asthma management.

How to Use the Right Inhaler Before Exercising

Using the correct inhaler before exercising is crucial for asthma patients to prevent symptoms. Generally, a rescue inhaler (usually containing albuterol) should be used approximately 15 to 30 minutes before physical activity. Make sure to shake the inhaler well, breathe out fully, and then inhale deeply while pressing down on the inhaler to release the medication.

After using the inhaler, hold your breath for about 10 seconds before exhaling to ensure the medication reaches the lungs effectively. This practice helps minimize the risk of exercise-induced asthma symptoms and enables a more comfortable workout.

Tips for Exercising in Different Weather Conditions

Weather can significantly impact asthma symptoms during exercise, so it's essential to take precautions. On cold days, warm up indoors and consider wearing a scarf or mask over the mouth to help warm the air before it enters your lungs. If exercising in hot and humid conditions, ensure proper hydration and consider exercising during cooler times of the day to avoid overheating, which can exacerbate symptoms.

If pollen levels are high, opt for indoor activities like gym workouts or swimming. Monitoring weather reports and pollen counts can help in planning safer exercise sessions that minimize asthma triggers, ensuring a healthier and more enjoyable experience.

Understanding Exercise-Induced Bronchoconstriction

Exercise-induced bronchoconstriction (EIB) occurs when physical activity leads to the narrowing of the airways, resulting in asthma symptoms. It can happen during or after exercise and is often triggered by high-intensity activities or exposure to cold, dry air. Understanding EIB helps patients recognize the signs, such as coughing, wheezing, or shortness of breath, allowing for prompt management.

To mitigate EIB, asthma patients should warm up properly, use a bronchodilator as prescribed before exercise, and engage in lower-intensity activities initially. Consulting with a healthcare provider for tailored advice and treatment options can help manage this condition effectively.

Strategies for Indoor Exercise Options

Indoor exercise options can provide a controlled environment for asthma patients, reducing exposure to outdoor allergens and weather-related triggers. Activities such as using a treadmill, stationary cycling, or participating in group classes can be effective alternatives to outdoor workouts. Indoor swimming pools can also be a good choice, as the humid environment can be less irritating to the airways.

To create a consistent indoor routine, consider investing in basic equipment or joining a local gym that offers asthma-friendly classes. Setting achievable fitness goals and tracking progress can help maintain motivation and ensure regular exercise while managing asthma symptoms.

Finding Asthma-Friendly Sports and Activities

Selecting asthma-friendly sports and activities is essential for maintaining an active lifestyle while managing asthma. Low-impact sports such as swimming, cycling, or walking can be ideal as they generally pose a lower risk for triggering symptoms. Individual sports, like yoga or tai chi, can also be beneficial since they allow participants to control intensity and duration.

When exploring new activities, communicate your asthma condition with instructors or coaches, who can provide modifications or alternatives. This proactive approach ensures safety and can help you enjoy the chosen sport without the worry of exacerbating asthma symptoms.

The Importance of Consistent Routine

Establishing a consistent exercise routine is crucial for asthma management. Regular physical activity can improve lung function, decrease the severity of symptoms, and enhance overall well-being. Try to schedule workouts at the same time each day to create a habit, making it easier to incorporate exercise into your daily life.

Incorporating a variety of activities into your routine can keep things interesting while addressing different aspects of fitness. Aim for a mix of cardiovascular, strength, and flexibility exercises to promote a well-rounded fitness regimen that supports lung health and reduces asthma symptoms.

Incorporating Stretching and Flexibility Exercises

Stretching and flexibility exercises play a significant role in overall fitness and can be particularly beneficial for asthma patients. These exercises help improve lung capacity and increase blood flow to the muscles, promoting better performance during physical activities. Incorporate dynamic stretches during your warm-up and static stretches during your cool-down to enhance flexibility and prevent injuries.

Incorporating yoga or Pilates can also be advantageous, as they combine stretching with controlled breathing techniques that promote relaxation and lung health. Aim to include stretching routines several times a week to maintain flexibility and support asthma management.

Role of Physical Therapy in Asthma Management

Physical therapy can play a vital role in asthma management by helping patients improve lung function and overall fitness levels. A physical therapist can design a personalized exercise program that accommodates individual asthma triggers and symptoms. This approach focuses on building endurance and strength while teaching effective breathing techniques.

Regular sessions with a physical therapist can help patients learn how to manage their asthma during exercise, monitor their symptoms, and adjust their routines accordingly.

Monitoring Symptoms During and After Exercise

Monitoring asthma symptoms during and after exercise is crucial for effective management. Keep a journal to track any symptoms experienced during physical activity, noting the type of exercise, intensity, and environmental conditions. This record can help identify patterns and triggers, allowing for more informed decisions about future workouts.

Post-exercise, assess your breathing and overall condition. If symptoms arise, use a rescue inhaler as needed, and consider consulting with a healthcare provider for further evaluation and potential adjustments to your asthma management plan. Regular monitoring ensures better control over symptoms and enhances overall exercise safety.

CHAPTER 8:

Managing Asthma in Children

Signs and Symptoms of Asthma in Children

Asthma symptoms in children can manifest in various ways, including persistent coughing, especially at night or during play, wheezing, shortness of breath, and chest tightness. Parents should be alert to changes in their child's breathing patterns or increased fatigue during physical activities, as these can indicate an asthma episode. Regularly monitoring these signs can help in early identification and management of the condition.

To effectively recognize asthma symptoms, keep a diary of your child's respiratory patterns and any triggers that may lead to attacks, such as allergens, weather changes, or physical exertion. This documentation can be invaluable for discussions with healthcare providers, aiding in tailoring treatment plans to better suit your child's specific needs.

Importance of Early Diagnosis and Treatment

Early diagnosis of asthma is crucial as it allows for timely intervention, reducing the risk of severe attacks and long-term complications. A healthcare provider will assess your child's symptoms, medical history, and may conduct tests like spirometry to confirm asthma. Starting treatment early can help manage symptoms more effectively and improve your child's overall quality of life.

Once diagnosed, a personalized asthma management plan should be developed, incorporating both medication and lifestyle adjustments. Regular follow-ups with your child's healthcare provider are essential to adjust the plan as needed, ensuring that the treatment remains effective and relevant to your child's changing needs.

Creating an Asthma-Friendly School Environment

To create an asthma-friendly school environment, it's vital to communicate with school administrators and staff about your child's condition. Provide a copy of their asthma action plan to teachers, school nurses, and any relevant staff members to ensure they understand how to respond during an asthma attack and how to help manage triggers in the classroom.

Schools can implement strategies such as keeping the environment free of dust and allergens, ensuring proper ventilation, and allowing access to medications as needed. Encouraging outdoor activities in less polluted areas and designating smoke-free zones will also contribute to a healthier environment for asthmatic children.

Teaching Children How to Manage Their Asthma

Teaching children to manage their asthma involves educating them about their condition, including recognizing symptoms and triggers. Children should be guided on how to use inhalers or nebulizers correctly, as well as the importance of adhering to their medication schedule. Engaging them in role-playing scenarios can enhance their understanding and comfort with managing their asthma.

Encourage children to advocate for themselves by explaining their condition to peers and teachers. This empowerment helps them feel more in control and reduces anxiety related to their asthma. Regular discussions about their experiences and any concerns can further reinforce their confidence in managing their health.

The Role of Caregivers in Asthma Management

Caregivers play a crucial role in managing a child's asthma by ensuring that the child adheres to their asthma action plan. This includes administering medications on time, recognizing early signs of an asthma attack, and helping the child avoid known triggers. Caregivers should also maintain open lines of communication with healthcare providers for ongoing support and guidance.

It's important for caregivers to model healthy behaviors, such as avoiding smoking or exposure to secondhand smoke, which can worsen asthma symptoms. Being proactive about managing the environment at home and school will help create a safer space for the child, contributing to better overall asthma management.

Common Challenges in Child Asthma Management

Common challenges in managing childhood asthma include inconsistent medication adherence, difficulties in recognizing symptoms, and the fear of physical activities. Children may forget to take their medications or may not understand the importance of their treatment, leading to increased risk of asthma attacks. It's essential to address these barriers through education and support.

To overcome these challenges, establish a routine for taking medications and create a reward system to encourage adherence. Engage children in discussions about their fears or hesitations regarding sports and activities, and reassure them that asthma does not have to limit their participation.

Communicating with Teachers and Caregivers

Effective communication with teachers and caregivers is essential for managing a child's asthma. Parents should provide teachers with a clear asthma action plan that outlines symptoms, triggers, and emergency procedures. Regular meetings or check-ins with educators can help ensure they are aware of any changes in the child's condition or treatment.

Encourage a collaborative approach by inviting teachers to ask questions and express any concerns they may have. This open dialogue helps build a supportive network around the child, allowing for timely interventions and ensuring that the child's needs are met both at school and at home.

Importance of Regular Check-Ups and Monitoring

Regular check-ups with a healthcare provider are crucial for monitoring a child's asthma and adjusting treatment as necessary. These visits allow for the assessment of lung function, a review of symptoms, and the effectiveness of current medications. Keeping a schedule of these appointments can help ensure that management remains proactive rather than reactive.

Parents should also utilize peak flow meters at home to track their child's lung function. Recording these measurements can provide valuable insights into the child's condition, enabling timely adjustments to their treatment plan and helping to prevent severe asthma episodes.

Resources for Children and Parents

Numerous resources are available for children and parents dealing with asthma. Organizations such as the American Lung Association provide educational materials, support groups, and advocacy tools to help families navigate asthma management. Local health departments may also offer workshops and resources tailored to asthma education.

Additionally, online forums and community support groups can connect families facing similar challenges. Sharing experiences and solutions with others can provide encouragement and practical tips that enhance asthma management at home and in the community.

Coping Strategies for Children during Asthma Attacks

Children can utilize various coping strategies during asthma attacks, including staying calm, using their prescribed inhaler, and practicing deep-breathing techniques. Encouraging children to identify a quiet space where they can rest and use their inhaler can also be beneficial. Teaching them to visualize calming scenes may help reduce anxiety during an attack.

Practicing these strategies in a controlled setting can prepare children for real-life situations. Role-playing can be particularly effective, allowing them to gain confidence in managing their symptoms independently while understanding the importance of seeking help when necessary.

Encouraging Children to Participate in Sports

Encouraging children with asthma to participate in sports is important for their physical and emotional well-being. It's essential to choose activities that are less likely to trigger asthma symptoms, such as swimming, cycling, or yoga. Work with a healthcare provider to create an individualized exercise plan that incorporates proper warm-up and cool-down routines.

Communicating with coaches and teammates about the child's asthma is key to ensuring their safety during activities. Educating them on how to support their friend during an asthma episode helps create a supportive environment where the child can participate confidently.

Educating Siblings about Asthma

Educating siblings about asthma fosters understanding and support within the family. Discussing the condition in an age-appropriate manner helps siblings grasp what asthma is, its symptoms, and how they can help during an asthma episode. This knowledge encourages empathy and reduces the likelihood of misunderstandings or fear related to their sibling's condition.

Involving siblings in asthma management, such as reminding their brother or sister to take their medication, can help them feel included and responsible. Family discussions about asthma can further strengthen bonds and create a supportive atmosphere where everyone is informed and engaged.

Support Networks for Families

Building a support network for families managing asthma is crucial for sharing experiences and gaining advice. Connecting with local or online support groups can provide valuable resources, emotional support, and practical tips for coping with the challenges of asthma management. Many organizations offer forums where families can ask questions and share their stories.

Additionally, parents should consider reaching out to healthcare providers for recommendations on local support services or community resources. These connections can enhance the family's understanding of asthma and provide ongoing support, ensuring that both children and parents feel empowered in their asthma journey.

CHAPTER 9:

Coping with Asthma

Emotional Impact of Living with Asthma

Living with asthma can significantly affect emotional well-being. Many individuals experience feelings of fear and anxiety related to their symptoms, especially during an asthma attack. The uncertainty of when an attack might occur can lead to stress and even avoidance of certain activities, impacting overall quality of life. It's important to recognize these emotions and understand that they are common among those managing this chronic condition.

To cope with the emotional toll, individuals can benefit from expressing their feelings and discussing their experiences with others. Engaging in regular physical activity, as approved by a healthcare provider, can also help alleviate some of the emotional burdens by releasing endorphins that promote a positive mood.

Practicing relaxation techniques, such as deep breathing exercises or mindfulness, can further assist in managing stress levels and improving emotional resilience.

Importance of Mental Health Support

Mental health support plays a crucial role in effectively managing asthma. The challenges associated with living with a chronic condition can lead to depression, anxiety, and social withdrawal. Seeking professional help from a therapist or counselor can provide valuable tools for coping with these feelings and can facilitate a more positive outlook on life with asthma.

Additionally, integrating mental health support into asthma management involves open communication with healthcare providers. They can help identify when emotional support is needed and recommend resources, such as support groups or therapy, tailored to individual needs. This collaboration fosters a holistic approach to health, ensuring that both physical and emotional aspects are addressed.

Strategies for Coping with Anxiety and Stress

Coping with anxiety and stress related to asthma involves implementing practical strategies that can be easily integrated into daily life. One effective approach is to create a personalized action plan that outlines steps to take during an asthma episode, which can help reduce feelings of helplessness. Regular physical activity and relaxation exercises, such as yoga or meditation, can also effectively lower stress levels and improve overall mental well-being.

In addition to these strategies, utilizing breathing techniques can help manage acute anxiety. For instance, practicing slow, deep breaths can calm the nervous system and alleviate feelings of panic during an asthma attack. Incorporating these techniques into daily routines allows individuals to feel more in control and can lead to better management of both asthma symptoms and emotional health.

The Role of Support Groups and Counseling

Support groups offer a valuable resource for individuals living with asthma, providing a platform to share experiences and strategies for managing the condition. Connecting with others who face similar challenges fosters a sense of community and reduces feelings of isolation. These groups can also provide practical tips for navigating everyday life with asthma, from managing triggers to dealing with emergencies.

Counseling, whether in individual or group settings, further enhances emotional support. A trained professional can help individuals explore their feelings about asthma and develop coping strategies tailored to their specific needs. Engaging in counseling can lead to increased self-acceptance and improved mental health, allowing individuals to approach their condition with confidence.

Techniques for Staying Positive and Motivated

Staying positive and motivated while managing asthma involves cultivating a mindset focused on possibilities rather than limitations. Setting small, achievable goals can provide a sense of accomplishment and encourage individuals to remain engaged in their treatment plans. Celebrating these small victories—like successfully completing a workout or managing symptoms during a stressful situation—reinforces positive behavior and fosters motivation.

Incorporating daily affirmations or mindfulness practices can also help maintain a positive outlook. These techniques encourage individuals to focus on their strengths and resilience, counteracting negative thoughts. By surrounding themselves with uplifting influences and maintaining a hopeful perspective, individuals can better navigate the challenges associated with asthma.

Importance of Education for Empowerment

Education is vital for empowering individuals to manage their asthma effectively. Understanding the condition—its triggers, symptoms, and treatment options—enables individuals to make informed decisions about their health. This knowledge fosters a sense of control and confidence, which is crucial for effective asthma management.

Additionally, educating oneself about asthma can lead to better communication with healthcare providers. Being well-informed allows patients to ask relevant questions, voice concerns, and participate actively in their treatment plans. Empowerment through education ultimately contributes to improved health outcomes and enhances quality of life for individuals living with asthma.

Building a Supportive Network of Friends and Family

Creating a supportive network of friends and family can significantly enhance emotional well-being for those living with asthma. Educating loved ones about the condition ensures they understand how to provide assistance during an asthma attack and can help minimize triggers in shared spaces. Open communication about needs and concerns fosters a supportive environment where individuals feel comfortable discussing their experiences.

Moreover, involving friends and family in lifestyle changes—such as exercising together or preparing asthma-friendly meals—can strengthen relationships and improve adherence to asthma management plans. This collective approach not only provides practical support but also nurtures a sense of belonging and understanding, making it easier for individuals to cope with the challenges of asthma.

Recognizing and Addressing Feelings of Isolation

Feelings of isolation are common among individuals living with asthma, particularly if they feel misunderstood or unsupported. Recognizing these emotions is the first step toward addressing them. Engaging in conversations with healthcare providers, friends, or support groups can provide validation and encourage individuals to share their experiences openly.

To combat feelings of isolation, individuals can explore activities that connect them with others, such as joining community classes or online forums dedicated to asthma support. Sharing experiences and challenges with others can help individuals realize they are not alone, fostering a sense of community and connection that is crucial for emotional health.

Setting Realistic Goals for Asthma Management

Setting realistic goals is essential for effective asthma management. Individuals should focus on attainable objectives that consider their unique circumstances and limitations. For example, rather than aiming to run a marathon immediately, one might start with short walks or gentle exercises that gradually increase in intensity.

Regularly revisiting and adjusting these goals as progress is made is equally important. Celebrating milestones, no matter how small, reinforces positive behaviors and motivates individuals to continue striving for better management. This practical approach allows individuals to maintain a balanced perspective and encourages sustained efforts toward health improvements.

Journaling as a Coping Mechanism

Journaling serves as an effective coping mechanism for individuals managing asthma. Writing about daily experiences, symptoms, and emotions can provide clarity and help process feelings associated with living with a chronic condition. This practice allows individuals to track patterns related to triggers and symptoms, facilitating better communication with healthcare providers.

In addition, journaling can act as a therapeutic outlet, enabling individuals to express frustrations, fears, and triumphs without judgment. Reflecting on written experiences fosters personal growth and can cultivate a more positive outlook, making it easier to cope with the challenges that asthma presents.

How to Celebrate Small Victories in Management

Celebrating small victories is a vital component of managing asthma and enhancing overall motivation. Acknowledging achievements—like successfully avoiding triggers during a stressful week or consistently taking medications—reinforces positive behavior and encourages continued commitment to management plans. Individuals can celebrate these moments by rewarding themselves with small treats or engaging in enjoyable activities.

Incorporating a visual reminder, such as a victory jar filled with notes of accomplishments, can also serve as a motivational tool. This tangible representation of progress can inspire individuals to maintain their efforts and remind them of their capabilities, fostering a positive mindset that encourages ongoing management success.

Sharing Your Story with Others for Support

Sharing personal experiences related to asthma can be a powerful way to gain support and foster connection. Individuals can benefit from discussing their journey with friends, family, or even in support groups. This openness can alleviate feelings of isolation and create opportunities for mutual understanding and empathy among those affected by asthma.

Moreover, sharing one's story can inspire others who may be struggling with similar challenges. By articulating both the difficulties and successes of managing asthma, individuals can empower others to seek help, pursue education, and foster their own support networks, ultimately creating a community of resilience and hope.

Embracing a Proactive Approach to Living with Asthma

Embracing a proactive approach to asthma management involves taking charge of one's health by actively engaging in prevention and treatment strategies. This includes regularly reviewing and updating an asthma action plan, understanding triggers, and adhering to prescribed medications. Individuals can also work closely with healthcare providers to set achievable health goals and monitor progress.

Furthermore, incorporating lifestyle changes—such as regular exercise, a balanced diet, and stress-reduction techniques—can significantly enhance asthma management. By adopting this proactive mindset, individuals can empower themselves to lead fulfilling lives while effectively managing their asthma symptoms and reducing the likelihood of attacks.

Common Concerns

Can Asthma Be Cured?

Currently, asthma cannot be cured, but it can be effectively managed. Understanding that asthma is a chronic condition means that while it might not go away completely, many people find ways to control their symptoms and lead active lives. Treatments include medications, lifestyle adjustments, and avoiding triggers that can worsen the condition.

To manage asthma, it's essential to work closely with your healthcare provider to develop a personalized asthma action plan. This plan outlines your medications, how to recognize worsening symptoms, and strategies for dealing with triggers, ensuring you have a clear path to follow for daily management.

What Should I Do During an Asthma Attack?

During an asthma attack, remain calm and try to find a comfortable position, typically sitting upright, which can help make breathing easier. Use your rescue inhaler as prescribed; this quick-relief medication can alleviate symptoms like wheezing, coughing, and shortness of breath within minutes. It's crucial to follow your asthma action plan and administer the medication according to your doctor's instructions.

If symptoms do not improve after using your inhaler, seek medical help immediately. This could involve calling emergency services or visiting the nearest hospital, especially if you experience severe difficulty breathing, chest tightness, or persistent symptoms despite medication.

Are There Any Dietary Restrictions?

While there are no strict dietary restrictions for asthma, certain foods may act as triggers for some individuals. Common culprits include sulfites (found in dried fruits and wine), dairy products, and foods high in trans fats. It's beneficial to keep a food diary to track what you eat and how it affects your symptoms, helping you identify potential triggers.

Incorporating anti-inflammatory foods into your diet can also be helpful. Focus on fruits, vegetables, whole grains, and healthy fats, such as omega-3 fatty acids found in fish and flaxseeds, which may help reduce inflammation in your airways.

How Often Should I See My Doctor?

Regular check-ups with your healthcare provider are vital for effective asthma management. Generally, it's recommended to see your doctor at least every six months or more frequently if your symptoms are not well-controlled or if you've recently experienced an asthma attack. These appointments help evaluate your condition and adjust your asthma action plan as needed.

In addition to regular visits, don't hesitate to contact your doctor if you notice any changes in your symptoms or if you have questions about your treatment. Open communication ensures that your management plan remains effective and tailored to your current needs.

What If My Medication Isn't Working?

If you find that your asthma medication isn't providing the relief you need, it's essential to consult your healthcare provider. They can review your current treatment plan and may suggest adjustments, such as changing dosages or trying a different medication altogether. Never adjust your medication without guidance from your doctor.

Additionally, ensure you're using your inhalers correctly. Sometimes, improper technique can lead to decreased effectiveness. Your doctor or a pharmacist can provide demonstrations and check your technique to ensure you're getting the full benefit of your medication.

Can I Exercise If I Have Asthma?

Yes, you can exercise with asthma, and physical activity can actually benefit your overall health. However, it's crucial to choose appropriate exercises and take precautions. Activities such as swimming, walking, or cycling are often well-tolerated and can help strengthen your lungs.

Before exercising, ensure your asthma is well-managed, and consider warming up beforehand. Keep your rescue inhaler nearby and take it as a preventive measure if recommended by your doctor. Monitor how your body responds during and after exercise to identify any triggers or patterns that may arise.

How Can I Help My Child Manage Asthma?

To help your child manage asthma effectively, start by educating them about their condition. Teach them how to recognize their symptoms and when to use their inhaler. Create an asthma action plan together, so they understand what to do in various situations, reinforcing their ability to advocate for their health.

Additionally, maintain a supportive environment at home and school. Ensure that teachers and caregivers know about your child's asthma and understand how to respond in case of an attack. Encourage regular medical check-ups and healthy lifestyle choices to support their overall well-being.

What Are the Long-Term Effects of Asthma?

The long-term effects of asthma can vary widely among individuals. If poorly managed, asthma can lead to persistent airway inflammation and remodeling, which may cause lasting breathing difficulties and reduced lung function. However, with proper management, many people can maintain good lung health and quality of life.

Monitoring and treating asthma effectively can prevent complications such as frequent hospitalizations and respiratory infections. Regular consultations with your healthcare provider help track your lung function and adjust your treatment plan to minimize long-term impacts.

Is It Safe to Take Multiple Medications?

In many cases, it is safe to take multiple medications for asthma, especially if prescribed by your healthcare provider. Often, a combination of long-term control medications and quick-relief inhalers is necessary for optimal management. Always follow your doctor's instructions regarding dosage and timing.

Keep an organized medication schedule to avoid missed doses and to track when you need to take each medication. Regularly review your medications with your healthcare provider to ensure they are still appropriate and effective for your condition.

How Do I Handle Asthma in Different Seasons?

Managing asthma during different seasons involves being aware of specific triggers associated with each time of year. In spring and summer, pollen can be a significant trigger, so consider staying indoors during high pollen counts and using air conditioning. Fall may bring dust and mold, while winter often introduces cold air as a potential trigger; wearing a scarf over your mouth and nose can help warm the air you breathe.

Keep your home environment as allergen-free as possible. Regularly clean and dust your living spaces, and consider using air purifiers to reduce indoor allergens. Staying informed about seasonal changes and potential triggers can help you adjust your asthma management strategies accordingly.

Frequently Asked Questions (FAQs)

What Is Asthma?

Asthma is a chronic respiratory condition characterized by inflammation of the airways, leading to difficulty breathing. Symptoms often include wheezing, shortness of breath, chest tightness, and coughing. These symptoms can vary in frequency and intensity among individuals.

Diagnosis typically involves a physical exam, medical history, and lung function tests. Understanding asthma as a lifelong condition allows for better management and symptom control.

What Causes Asthma?

Asthma triggers can vary from person to person and may include allergens, respiratory infections, exercise, cold air, and smoke. Genetic factors also play a role, as asthma often runs in families. Identifying and avoiding personal triggers is essential for effective asthma management.

Environmental factors, such as pollution and occupational exposures, can contribute to the development of asthma or exacerbate symptoms. Awareness of these influences can help individuals take proactive steps to reduce their impact.

How Do I Know If I Have Asthma?

Common signs of asthma include recurrent episodes of wheezing, coughing, chest tightness, and difficulty breathing, especially at night or early in the morning. If you experience these symptoms frequently, it's essential to consult a healthcare professional for an evaluation.

Diagnostic tests, such as spirometry, can help determine if asthma is present by measuring how much air you can exhale and how quickly. A thorough assessment will help identify whether asthma is the cause of your symptoms.

What Should I Do If I Experience Asthma Symptoms?

If you experience asthma symptoms, first use your rescue inhaler as prescribed. Try to remain calm and assess your situation—sometimes, symptoms may improve with controlled breathing techniques. Keeping a diary of your symptoms can help you and your doctor understand when and why they occur.

If your symptoms do not improve after using your inhaler, seek medical attention. Knowing when to escalate your care can prevent severe complications and ensure timely treatment.

Are There Specific Medications for Asthma?

Yes, there are several medications specifically designed for asthma management. Long-term control medications, such as inhaled corticosteroids and leukotriene modifiers, help reduce inflammation and prevent symptoms. Quick-relief inhalers provide fast relief during asthma attacks.

Consult your healthcare provider to determine the best medication plan for your needs, as individual responses to treatments can vary. Regularly review your medications and dosages to ensure they remain effective.

How Can I Identify My Asthma Triggers?

Identifying asthma triggers involves careful observation of your environment and symptoms. Keeping a detailed journal can help track when symptoms occur and what factors may have contributed, such as weather changes, allergens, or stress levels.

Common triggers include dust mites, pet dander, mold, pollen, and smoke. Once identified, take steps to reduce exposure, such as cleaning regularly and avoiding known allergens.

What Lifestyle Changes Can Improve Asthma?

Making certain lifestyle changes can significantly improve asthma management. Quitting smoking and avoiding secondhand smoke are crucial for reducing symptoms. Regular physical activity, when done safely, can help strengthen your lungs and improve overall fitness.

Additionally, maintaining a healthy diet, managing stress, and ensuring adequate sleep can support better respiratory health. These holistic approaches can enhance your quality of life while managing asthma effectively.

Is It Safe to Use Inhalers Frequently?

Using inhalers as prescribed by your healthcare provider is generally safe. However, reliance on quick-relief inhalers may indicate that your asthma is not well-controlled. If you find yourself using your inhaler more than twice a week, consult your doctor for an evaluation and possible adjustments to your treatment plan.

Proper inhaler technique is also essential to ensure you receive the full benefit of your medication. Ask your healthcare provider for a demonstration if you're unsure about how to use your inhaler correctly.

What Are the Differences Between Asthma and Allergies?

Asthma and allergies are related but distinct conditions. Asthma is primarily a respiratory issue characterized by difficulty breathing, while allergies involve the immune system reacting to specific substances (allergens). Many people with asthma also have allergies, which can exacerbate their symptoms.

Identifying whether you are experiencing asthma or allergy symptoms is crucial for effective management. Treatment may involve medications for asthma control as well as antihistamines or other therapies for allergy relief.

Conclusion

Creating an Asthma Action Plan

An asthma action plan is a written plan developed with your healthcare provider that outlines your asthma management strategies, including medication dosages, trigger avoidance, and emergency steps to take during an asthma attack. Work together with your doctor to create a personalized action plan that fits your lifestyle and specific asthma needs.

Review and update your asthma action plan regularly, especially after any changes in your symptoms or treatment. Having a clear plan helps you stay organized and empowers you to manage your asthma more effectively, providing peace of mind during unexpected situations.

Breathing Techniques

Breathing techniques, such as pursed-lip breathing and diaphragmatic breathing, can help you manage asthma symptoms effectively. Pursed-lip breathing involves inhaling through the nose and exhaling slowly through pursed lips, which can help keep airways open longer and make breathing easier. Diaphragmatic breathing focuses on engaging the diaphragm, allowing for deeper breaths that can improve oxygen exchange.

To practice these techniques, find a quiet space to focus on your breathing. Start by inhaling deeply and exhaling slowly, aiming to increase the length of your exhales. Regular practice can enhance your ability to control your breathing during asthma attacks and improve overall lung function.

Avoiding Allergens and Irritants

Reducing exposure to allergens and irritants is crucial for asthma management. Common allergens include dust mites, mold, pet dander, and pollen. To minimize exposure, consider using HEPA filters in your home, regularly washing bedding in hot water, and keeping windows closed during high pollen seasons.

Irritants like smoke, strong odors, and pollution can also trigger asthma symptoms. Avoid smoking and stay away from secondhand smoke, and limit exposure to strong chemical fumes. By proactively managing your environment, you can significantly reduce your asthma triggers and improve your quality of life.

Regular Check-ups

Regular check-ups with your healthcare provider are essential for effective asthma management. These appointments allow you to review your symptoms, medication effectiveness, and any necessary adjustments to your treatment plan. Staying consistent with your check-ups helps monitor your asthma's progression and ensures you are using the best strategies for control.

During these visits, openly communicate any changes in your symptoms or concerns about your treatment. Your healthcare provider can offer valuable insights and help you stay informed about the latest asthma management strategies, ensuring you have the tools needed for effective control.

Utilizing Technology

Technology can play a significant role in asthma management. Many apps are available to help track symptoms, medication usage, and triggers. These tools can provide reminders for taking medications and alerts about air quality and pollen levels, enabling you to make informed decisions about outdoor activities.

Additionally, smart inhalers equipped with sensors can help monitor medication usage and share data with your healthcare provider. Embracing technology in your asthma management can enhance your awareness and improve your ability to control your condition effectively.

Engaging in Physical Activity

Regular physical activity is essential for overall health and can help improve asthma control. While some may worry that exercise could trigger symptoms, many individuals with asthma can engage in sports and activities with the right precautions. Choose activities that suit your fitness level, and consider starting with lower-intensity exercises, gradually increasing intensity as your endurance improves.

Before exercising, be sure to warm up adequately, and keep your quick-relief inhaler on hand. If you experience symptoms during or after exercise, consult your healthcare provider to adjust your action plan. With proper management, you can enjoy the benefits of physical activity without compromising your asthma control.

Nutrition and Diet

A balanced diet rich in fruits, vegetables, whole grains, and healthy fats can support overall lung health and potentially reduce asthma symptoms. Foods rich in antioxidants, such as berries and leafy greens, may help lower inflammation, while omega-3 fatty acids found in fish can also have beneficial effects.

Staying hydrated is equally important, as dehydration can exacerbate asthma symptoms. Pay attention to any food sensitivities or allergies that may trigger symptoms and work with a nutritionist if needed to develop a tailored dietary plan that promotes better asthma management.

Stress Management

Stress can exacerbate asthma symptoms, making stress management a vital aspect of your overall treatment plan. Techniques such as mindfulness, meditation, and yoga can help reduce stress levels and improve breathing control. Consider incorporating these practices into your daily routine to promote relaxation and enhance your ability to cope with asthma.

Additionally, seek support from friends, family, or support groups to share your experiences and learn from others facing similar challenges. By managing stress effectively, you can create a more supportive environment for your asthma management and improve your overall well-being.

Ongoing Education and Support

Staying informed about asthma and its management is crucial for success. Participate in educational programs, attend workshops, or read up-to-date literature to deepen your understanding of asthma. Knowledge empowers you to recognize symptoms, manage triggers, and communicate effectively with your healthcare provider.

Moreover, joining support groups or online forums can provide valuable emotional support and practical advice from those with similar experiences. Engaging in ongoing education and seeking community support can significantly enhance your asthma management journey, making it a shared experience rather than a solitary struggle.